Revitalize Your Health

A Comprehensive Guide to Boosting Metabolism, Shedding Fat, and Extending Your Lifespan

JULIAN TIM

Table of Contents

The Sleep Solution for Optimal Health Everyday Habits for Disease Defense and Longevity

Conclusion

Introduction

In the dynamic tapestry of life, our well-being is a crucial thread that we weave through the choices we make each day. This book is an empowering journey into the realms of metabolism, fat loss, and longevity, offering you a roadmap to transform your health and vitality.

In these pages, we will delve into the intricate mechanisms of metabolism, unlocking the secrets to enhancing your body's natural ability to burn energy efficiently. You'll discover practical strategies for shedding excess fat, backed by scientific insights and sustainable lifestyle adjustments. Moreover, we'll explore the fascinating science behind extending your lifespan, embracing a holistic approach that encompasses not just years added to life but life added to years.

Whether you are starting on a wellness journey or seeking to revitalize your existing health routine, this guide is tailored to meet you where you are. With evidence-based advice, actionable tips, and a focus on personalized well-being, "Revitalize Your Health" is more than a book – it's a companion on your path to a healthier, more vibrant you. Embark on this transformative adventure, and let the pages ahead be the catalyst for a renewed sense of vitality, longevity, and a profound connection to the best version of yourself.

Now is the moment to take charge of your health journey. "Revitalize Your Health" is not just a guide; it's your ticket to a revitalized and empowered life. The transformative insights within these pages are waiting to be applied, and the sooner you embrace them, the sooner you unlock the doors to a healthier, more vibrant you. Imagine the energy, the confidence, and the longevity that lie ahead. Don't let this opportunity slip away. Click that order button, dive into the wealth of knowledge that awaits you, and let "Revitalize Your Health" be the catalyst for a journey that will reshape your well-being. Your body deserves the best care, and the time to start is now. Your revitalized life begins with a single step—make it now.

Chapter One
Understanding metabolism for a Healthier You

Understanding metabolism is like grasping how your body transforms the food you eat into energy to fuel all your daily activities. Think of it as a busy factory inside you, breaking down food (catabolism) to make energy and building essential substances (anabolism) your body needs. Your metabolic rate is like the factory's speed, and things like exercising, eating well, and sleeping enough can influence how fast or slow it works.

Imagine your body as a smart manager making decisions on how to use the resources (food) efficiently. Some foods provide quick energy, while others are stored for later. It's not just about counting calories; it's about understanding which foods support your energy needs.

Metabolism can be broadly divided into two main components: anabolism and catabolism. Anabolism involves building and repairing tissues, such as muscle growth, while catabolism breaks down substances to release energy. Striking a balance between these processes is key to a well-functioning metabolism.

Your metabolic rate is the speed at which your body burns calories. It's influenced by factors like genetics, age, gender, and muscle mass. While some of these factors are beyond your control, there are practical steps you can take to boost your metabolism and optimize your overall health.

Factors Affecting Metabolism

1. **Genetics:** Your genetic makeup plays a role in determining your baseline metabolic rate. While you can't change your genes, understanding them can help you make informed choices for a healthier lifestyle.
2. **Age:** Metabolism tends to slow down with age, primarily due to a decrease in muscle mass. Engaging in regular physical activity

and maintaining a balanced diet become even more crucial as you age.

3. **Gender:** Generally the metabolic rate in men is more than that of women. However, factors like body composition and hormonal fluctuations can impact metabolism differently for each individual.

4. **Muscle Mass:** Muscles burn more calories at rest than fat. Incorporating strength training into your exercise routine can help build and maintain muscle, contributing to a higher metabolic rate.

5. **Nutrition:** What and how you eat significantly influences your metabolism. Consuming a balanced diet with an appropriate mix of proteins, carbohydrates, and fats supports your body's energy needs.

Revitalizing your health

Revitalizing your health is crucial for overall well-being and a fulfilling life. Firstly, physical health plays a fundamental role in our daily activities. When you prioritize exercise, nutritious eating, and sufficient sleep, you enhance your body's functionality, promoting better energy levels and a more robust immune system. This, in turn, allows you to engage more actively in work, hobbies, and relationships.

Secondly, mental health is intrinsically linked to overall vitality. Stress, anxiety, and other mental health challenges can significantly impact physical well-being. Taking steps to revitalize your mental health, such as practicing mindfulness or seeking support when needed, contributes to a more balanced and resilient mind. A healthy mind not only copes better with life's challenges but also positively influences decision-making and emotional well-being.

Furthermore, revitalizing your health has long-term benefits, reducing the risk of chronic diseases and enhancing longevity. Healthy lifestyle choices, including regular exercise and a balanced diet, contribute to maintaining optimal weight and preventing conditions like heart disease, diabetes, and hypertension. By investing in your health now, you are laying the foundation for a more vibrant and active future.

Lastly, the importance of revitalizing your health extends beyond the individual level. When individuals prioritize their well-being, it has a ripple effect on communities and societies. Healthier individuals are often more productive, contribute positively to their communities, and may inspire others to adopt healthier habits. Thus, revitalizing your health is not only a personal investment but also a contribution to the collective well-being of the larger community.

How to Revitalize Your Health

Improving your overall health involves adopting a holistic approach that encompasses physical, mental, and emotional well-being. Here are practical ways to revitalize your health:

Consume a balanced diet daily. Eat whole grains, vegetables, lean proteins and fruits. Limit processed foods, sugars, and unhealthy fats to support optimal bodily function. Also, engage in regular physical activity. Choose exercises you enjoy, whether it's brisk walking, cycling, swimming, or yoga. Aim for at least 150 minutes of moderate-intensity exercise per week, enhancing cardiovascular health and maintaining a healthy weight.

Sleep in a comfortable place and create a consistent sleep schedule. Quality sleep is crucial for overall well-being. Drinking enough water to maintain proper hydration is very imperative as this supports various functions in the body, such as circulation, regulation of temperature and food digestion.

Various relaxation techniques such as deep breathing, meditation, or mindfulness should be adopted in management of stress. Incorporate activities you find enjoyable to unwind, fostering a balanced emotional state.Establish a routine for regular health check-ups and screenings. Early detection of potential health issues allows for timely intervention, promoting long-term well-being.

Cultivate social connections by spending time with friends, family, and supportive communities. Strong social ties contribute to emotional resilience and can positively impact mental health. Limit alcohol intake and avoid tobacco products. These habits have detrimental effects on your physical health, increasing the risk of various diseases.

Proper hygiene as good oral care and regular hand washing should be maintained. Maintaining cleanliness supports the prevention of infections and contributes to overall health.Continuously educate yourself about health and wellness. Stay informed about current research, and consider consulting with healthcare professionals or nutritionists to tailor advice to your specific needs.

Above all, embrace a positive mindset. Be grateful, compassionate and set achievable goals. A positive outlook can significantly influence your overall health and quality of life.

Chapter Two

Nutritional Mastery for Health

Nutritional Mastery for Health encompasses the comprehensive understanding and proficient application of nutritional principles to achieve and maintain optimal well-being. It involves a deep knowledge of the role that various nutrients play in supporting the body's functions, including energy metabolism, immune system function, and cellular repair. Mastery in nutrition implies the ability to make informed choices about dietary habits, recognizing the impact of different foods on overall health and addressing individual nutritional needs.

Achieving "Nutritional Mastery for Health" goes beyond simply knowing nutritional facts; it involves the practical integration of this knowledge into daily life. This includes designing well-balanced and personalized meal plans, considering factors such as age, gender, activity level, and specific health goals. Individuals who attain nutritional mastery are adept at navigating the complex landscape of dietary advice, understanding the nuances of different diets, and making informed decisions that align with their unique health requirements.

Ultimately, "Nutritional Mastery for Health" empowers individuals to take control of their well-being through conscious and educated choices. It promotes a proactive approach to health, recognizing the intimate connection between nutrition and overall vitality. By mastering the principles of nutrition, individuals can optimize their dietary habits to enhance physical and mental health, fostering a holistic and sustainable foundation for well-rounded wellness.

Crafting Your Nutrient-Rich Plate.

The strategic approach to building a balanced and nourishing plate, serving as a cornerstone for overall well-being is clearly explained. The essence lies in selecting a variety of nutrient-dense foods that cater to individual nutritional needs. This involves a thoughtful combination of essential macronutrients such as proteins, carbohydrates, and healthy fats, alongside a rich assortment of micronutrients like vitamins and minerals.

The significance of crafting a nutrient-rich plate goes beyond mere sustenance; it is a proactive measure towards optimizing metabolism and promoting fat loss. The book underscores the idea that a plate abundant in diverse, whole foods not only fuels the body but also supports key metabolic functions. By focusing on nutrient density, readers are guided to make informed choices that contribute to sustained energy levels and vitality. The subtitle serves as a practical guide, providing readers with actionable steps to transform their dietary habits, fostering a positive impact on their overall health.

In essence, "Crafting Your Nutrient-Rich Plate" encapsulates the philosophy of holistic health mastery presented in "Revitalize Your Health." It empowers readers to take control of their nutrition, offering a roadmap for designing meals that not only taste good but also serve as a catalyst for metabolic enhancement, fat loss, and the extension of a healthy lifespan. As readers delve into this aspect of health crafting, they are equipped with the tools to make intentional, health-promoting choices that resonate with the overarching theme of the book.

Understanding Nutrient Density

At the heart of crafting a nutrient-rich plate lies the concept of nutrient density. It's not just about the quantity of food but the quality of the nutrients it delivers. Begin by embracing a colorful spectrum of fruits and vegetables. These vibrant hues signify a diverse range of antioxidants, vitamins, and minerals essential for cellular function and metabolic efficiency. The goal is to maximize nutrient diversity on your plate, ensuring a robust intake of micronutrients that form the foundation of a thriving body.

Balancing Macronutrients:

Crafting a nutrient-rich plate involves a delicate dance of macronutrients – proteins, carbohydrates, and fats. Opt for lean proteins such as poultry, fish, or plant-based alternatives like legumes. Proteins are the building blocks of life, supporting muscle growth and repair. Complement this with whole grains, providing complex carbohydrates that sustain energy levels and contribute to a feeling of fullness. Incorporating healthy fats, sourced from avocados, nuts, and olive oil, not only adds a layer of satiety to your meals but also aids in the absorption of fat-soluble vitamins.

Portion Control and Mindful Eating:

Practicality in crafting your nutrient-rich plate extends to portion control and mindful eating. Recognize hunger and fullness cues to guide the quantity of food you consume. Consider subdividing your plate into sections, allocating space for different food groups. This visual aid can serve as a practical tool to ensure a balanced intake. Mindful eating encourages a conscious connection with the act of eating, fostering a healthier relationship with food and promoting a sense of satisfaction that goes beyond mere nourishment.

Fine-Tuning Your Nutrient-Rich Plate: Achieving Synergy

The Power of Plant-Based Foods:

Zooming in on the plant-based components of your plate, embrace the diversity of vegetables and fruits. Foods rich in fiber enhance digestive health and also make one full.Additionally, the myriad phytonutrients present in fruits and vegetables act as antioxidants, combating oxidative stress and inflammation within the body.

Proteins for Muscle Health:

In the realm of proteins, the focus extends beyond quantity to quality. Opt for lean sources that provide essential amino acids vital for muscle health.

Whether it's lean poultry, fatty fish rich in omega-3 fatty acids, or plant-based proteins like beans and lentils, the goal is to integrate diverse protein sources into your diet. This not only supports muscle maintenance but also facilitates the repair processes crucial for overall well-being.

Complex Carbs for Sustained Energy:

Whole grains take center stage as the source of complex carbohydrates in your nutrient-rich plate. These include options like quinoa, brown rice, and oats, offering sustained energy release. Unlike refined carbohydrates, which can lead to energy spikes and crashes, complex carbs provide a steady stream of energy, supporting both physical and cognitive functions.

Healthy Fats: The Balancing Act:

The inclusion of healthy fats is a critical aspect of achieving a balanced nutrient-rich plate. Avocados, nuts, seeds, and olive oil contribute not only to the flavor and satiety of your meals but also ensure the absorption of fat-soluble vitamins A, D, E, and K. Striking the right balance in fat intake is key – it's about embracing the health benefits of fats while being mindful of portion sizes.

Sustainability and Enjoyability: Making Nutrient-Rich Eating a Lifestyle

The Role of Sustainability:

Crafting a nutrient-rich plate is not just about short-term gains; it's about fostering a sustainable and enjoyable way of eating. Consider the environmental impact of your food choices by incorporating locally sourced and seasonal produce. This not only supports sustainable agriculture but also adds a layer of freshness and variety to your meals.

Incorporating Variety and Flexibility:

The journey to health through nutrient-rich plates is not a rigid path. Embrace variety and flexibility in your food choices. Consume varieties of fruits, vegetables, proteins, and grains. These make your meal enjoyable. This not only prevents dietary monotony but also ensures a broad spectrum of nutrients over time.

Mindful Indulgences:

Health crafting doesn't mean eliminating indulgences entirely. Allow yourself mindful indulgences from time to time. Whether it's a piece of dark chocolate or a small serving of your favorite treat, these occasional indulgences can be integrated into a nutrient-rich eating plan without compromising overall health goals.

Putting Knowledge into Practice: Crafting Your Nutrient-Rich Plate in Daily Life

Meal Planning for Success:

Practicality in crafting a nutrient-rich plate extends to meal planning. Take time to plan your meals, considering the nutritional content of each dish. This not only streamlines your grocery shopping but also ensures that you have the necessary ingredients to create balanced and nutritious meals throughout the week.

Quick and Nutrient-Packed Recipes:

In a world where time is often a limiting factor, having a repertoire of quick and nutrient-packed recipes is invaluable. Explore simple yet nourishing recipes that align with your taste preferences and lifestyle. From smoothie bowls to one-pan meals, these recipes showcase that crafting a nutrient-rich plate can be both convenient and delicious.

Listening to Your Body:

Ultimately, the most practical guide to crafting your nutrient-rich plate lies within your own body. Watch out for how your body reacts to various kinds of food. Notice the energy levels, digestion, and overall well-being associated with various meals. This intuitive approach to eating allows you to fine-tune your nutrient-rich plate based on your unique needs and preferences.

Crafting Your Nutrient-Rich Plate for a Lifelong Journey

In the realm of health crafting, "Crafting Your Nutrient-Rich Plate" stands as a powerful and practical tool. It's a dynamic process that combines knowledge, variety, and mindful choices to create meals that not only support immediate health goals but also contribute to a resilient and vibrant life in the long run. As you embark on this journey, remember that crafting your nutrient-rich plate is a skill that evolves with time. It's about progress, not perfection, and the small, consistent choices you make each day culminate in a lifestyle that revitalizes your health, boosts metabolism, sheds fat, and extends your lifespan.

Superfoods and Their Fat-Burning Power

Foods packed with exceptional nutrients for the proper functioning of the body are referred to as Superfoods. When it comes to fat-burning, certain superfoods are often touted for their metabolism-boosting properties. Understanding the relationship between superfoods and their fat-burning power requires delving into the nutritional aspects that contribute to weight management.

One key group of superfoods known for their fat-burning potential is leafy greens. Vegetables like kale, spinach, and Swiss chard are rich in vitamins, minerals, and antioxidants. These nutrients support overall health and, indirectly, weight management. The high fiber content in leafy greens promotes satiety, helping individuals feel full and potentially reducing overall caloric intake. Additionally, antioxidants in these greens may contribute to a healthier metabolism, although the extent of their fat-burning impact is subject to ongoing research.

Berries, another category of superfoods, are celebrated not only for their delicious taste but also for their potential in aiding weight loss. Blueberries, raspberries, and strawberries are packed with antioxidants and fiber, which can contribute to a feeling of fullness and help regulate blood sugar levels. The natural sweetness of berries also makes them a satisfying alternative to sugary snacks, supporting efforts to reduce overall calorie consumption.

Fatty fish, such as salmon and mackerel, are rich in omega-3 fatty acids, which have been linked to various health benefits, including potential support for fat loss. Omega-3s may influence the body's metabolism, helping it burn fat more efficiently. Moreover, the protein content in fish contributes to a feeling of fullness, which can aid in weight management by reducing the likelihood of overeating.

Green tea, often considered a superfood beverage, contains catechins, which are antioxidants that may assist in boosting metabolism and enhancing fat burning. While the effects of green tea on weight loss are modest, incorporating it into a balanced diet and active lifestyle may provide additional support for those aiming to shed excess pounds.

It's crucial to note that while certain superfoods may have fat-burning properties, relying solely on them for weight loss is unrealistic. A holistic approach to health, including a well-balanced diet, regular physical activity, and adequate sleep, remains fundamental for achieving and maintaining a healthy weight.

Superfoods can play a role in supporting weight management through various mechanisms such as promoting satiety, regulating blood sugar levels, and enhancing metabolism. Leafy greens, berries, fatty fish, and green tea are among the superfoods recognized for their potential fat-burning power. However, incorporating these foods into a broader lifestyle approach that includes a balanced diet and regular exercise is essential for achieving sustainable and effective results in the pursuit of a healthy weight.

Chapter Three

Exercise Essentials for Vitality

This emphasizes a holistic approach to fitness, combining cardiovascular, strength, flexibility, and balance exercises to promote overall well-being. The program recognizes the interconnectedness of physical and mental health, incorporating activities that not only enhance physical fitness but also contribute to stress reduction and mental clarity. With a focus on consistency and variety, it encourages individuals to find activities they enjoy, fostering a sustainable and enjoyable fitness routine. Additionally, proper nutrition and adequate rest are integral components, reinforcing the idea that vitality is a result of comprehensive lifestyle choices rather than isolated workout sessions.

Tailored workouts are the key to achieving real and sustainable fitness results. Unlike generic exercise plans, tailored workouts are specifically crafted to suit individual needs, considering factors like fitness level, goals, and any existing limitations.

This personalized approach ensures that each exercise is purposeful and aligns with the individual's unique requirements.

Tailored Workouts for Real Results

The foundation of tailored workouts lies in a thorough understanding of the individual's fitness objectives. Whether the goal is weight loss, muscle gain, or overall health improvement, a tailored workout takes these aspirations into account, creating a roadmap for success. For instance, a program aiming for weight loss might incorporate a combination of cardio and strength training exercises to maximize calorie burn and enhance metabolism. One of the primary advantages of tailored workouts is efficiency. By focusing on exercises that directly contribute to the desired outcome, individuals can optimize their time spent in the gym. This targeted approach minimizes the risk of wasted effort on activities that don't align with the overarching fitness goals.

Furthermore, tailored workouts adapt to the individual's progress and changing needs. Regular assessments allow for adjustments to the workout plan, ensuring continued challenge and growth. This adaptability is crucial for preventing plateaus and keeping the body responsive to the training stimulus.

Tailored workouts also consider individual preferences and lifestyle factors. By incorporating activities that individuals enjoy, adherence to the exercise routine is more likely. This personalization makes the journey to fitness more enjoyable and sustainable in the long run.

Additionally, addressing any existing physical limitations or health concerns is paramount in a tailored workout plan. Modifications can be made to accommodate injuries or health conditions, ensuring a safe and effective fitness journey. This personalized approach minimizes the risk of exacerbating existing issues and promotes overall well-being.

Tailored workouts are the linchpin to achieving real and lasting fitness results. By customizing exercise plans to individual goals, preferences, and limitations, these workouts maximize efficiency, adapt to progress, and enhance overall well-being. Embracing a tailored approach is an investment in one's health, providing a roadmap to success that is both effective and sustainable.

High-Intensity Interval Training (HIIT): Unleash the Power of Intervals

HIIT is like the superhero of workouts. Instead of slogging through long, monotonous exercises, HIIT spices things up with short bursts of intense effort followed by brief rest periods. It's the cardio rebel that boosts your heart rate, burns calories, and leaves you feeling like you conquered Everest in just a few minutes.

Picture this: You sprint like Usain Bolt for 30 seconds, catching your breath for 15 seconds, and then repeat. This cycle of push and recovery is the magic of HIIT. It's not just about how long you sweat but how hard. HIIT is efficient, making it the ideal workout for busy bees who want results without spending hours at the gym.

Strength Training: Sculpt Your Powerhouse

Enter strength training, the muscle sculptor. While HIIT gets your heart racing, strength training hones in on building muscles. Forget the myth that lifting weights turns you into the Hulk. In reality, it's your ticket to a lean, strong body.

With strength training, you lift weights or use your body weight to challenge your muscles. Squats, deadlifts, push-ups – these are your tools. The magic lies in controlled movements, pushing your muscles to adapt and grow. Plus, muscles are like calorie-burning furnaces; the more you have, the more calories you torch, even at rest.

The Dynamic Duo: Unbeatable Tag Team

Now, imagine combining these powerhouses. HIIT and strength training, the dynamic duo. While HIIT torches fat and improves cardiovascular health, strength training shapes and defines your physique. Together, they're a force multiplier.

HIIT prepares the stage, revving up your metabolism and priming your body for action. Then comes strength training, sculpting your muscles with precision. It's the perfect synergy – HIIT for the heart and fat, strength training for the muscles and metabolism.

Why This Duo Rocks:

1. *Efficiency:* Say goodbye to long, tedious workouts. This duo delivers results in less time.
2. *Fat Burn Fiesta*: HIIT ignites the fat-burning furnace, while strength training keeps it roaring.

3. *Metabolic Boost*: Your body becomes a 24/7 calorie-burning machine, thanks to muscle gain and HIIT's afterburn effect.

The HIIT and strength training duo is your shortcut to a fit, strong, and energized self. It's not just a workout; it's a lifestyle upgrade. Dive in, break a sweat, and let the dynamic duo transform your fitness game!

Chapter Four

Stress-Free Living for Well-being

Stress-free living is a cornerstone of overall well-being, offering a pathway to a healthier and more fulfilling life. One key strategy involves cultivating mindfulness, which means staying present in the moment without judgment. This can be achieved through practices such as meditation or simply by focusing on your breath. By embracing mindfulness, you create a mental space that allows you to respond to challenges with clarity rather than reacting impulsively. This shift in perspective can significantly reduce stress, promoting a sense of calm and balance.

Another crucial aspect of stress-free living is establishing healthy boundaries. It's essential to recognize your limits and learn to say no when necessary. Prioritizing self-care, setting realistic goals, and maintaining a balanced lifestyle contribute to a more resilient and stress-resistant mindset. By incorporating these practices into your daily routine, you not only enhance your mental and emotional well-being but also empower yourself to navigate life's challenges with greater ease and confidence.

Mind-Body Harmony for Stress Reduction

In the fast-paced world we inhabit, stress has become an unwelcome companion for many. The intricate connection between the mind and body offers a powerful avenue for mitigating this stress. Mind-body harmony, rooted in practices like mindfulness and meditation, provides a practical and clear path toward stress reduction.

Understanding the Mind-Body Connection:

The mind and body are intricately intertwined, with each influencing the other in a dynamic dance. The issue of stress has both physical and mental implications. Recognizing this connection is the first step toward achieving harmony and balance.

Mindfulness Practices:

Mindfulness, a cornerstone of mind-body harmony, involves bringing one's attention to the present moment without judgment. Techniques such as deep breathing, body scans, and guided meditation serve as tools to anchor the mind in the present, breaking the cycle of stress-inducing thoughts.

Cultivating Awareness:

The mind often races ahead, dwelling on future uncertainties or lingering on past regrets. Mind-body harmony encourages cultivating awareness of these thought patterns. By acknowledging and gently redirecting the mind to the present moment, individuals can alleviate the mental burdens contributing to stress.

The Power of Breath:

A simple yet profound aspect of mind-body harmony is conscious breathing. Body's relaxation response is activated by deep, intentional breaths.

calming the nervous system. Incorporating practices like diaphragmatic breathing into daily routines provides a portable and accessible stress reduction tool.

Physical Activity as a Mind-Body Bridge:

Engaging in physical activity not only benefits the body but also nurtures the mind. Exercise releases endorphins, the body's natural mood lifters, while simultaneously promoting mental clarity. Whether through yoga, walking, or other forms of exercise, the integration of movement is a vital component of mind-body harmony.

Nutrition and Mind-Body Wellness:

The connection between nutrition and stress is often underestimated. A well-balanced diet, rich in nutrients, supports both physical and mental well-being. Mindful eating, paying attention to the flavors and textures of each bite, enhances the mind-body connection and fosters a sense of satisfaction.

Consistency and Patience:

Achieving mind-body harmony for stress reduction is a gradual process that requires consistency and patience. Like any skill, mindfulness and related practices strengthen with regularity. Setting realistic expectations and allowing oneself the grace to grow over time is integral to success.

Building Mental Resilience in Daily Life

Building mental resilience is crucial for navigating life's challenges. Here are practical ways to cultivate resilience in your daily routine:

1. Develop a Positive Mindset:

- Foster optimism by reframing negative thoughts.
- Practice gratitude to shift focus towards positive aspects of life.

2. Cultivate Strong Social Connections:

- Build a support network of friends and family.
- Nurture relationships through regular communication and shared activities.

3. Prioritize Self-Care:

- Ensure adequate sleep to support mental well-being.
- Incorporate regular exercise to reduce stress and enhance mood.

4. Embrace Change and Adaptability:

- View challenges as opportunities for growth.
- Develop flexibility by intentionally stepping out of comfort zones.

5. Set Realistic Goals:

- Break larger goals into smaller, achievable steps.
- Celebrate small victories to boost confidence and motivation.

6. Practice Mindfulness and Relaxation Techniques:

- Engage in meditation or deep-breathing exercises.
- Stay present in the moment to reduce anxiety about the future.

7. Learn Problem-Solving Skills:

- Approach problems analytically and break them down.
- Seek solutions rather than dwelling on obstacles.

8. Develop Emotional Intelligence:

- Understand and manage your emotions effectively.
- Empathize with others to build stronger connections.

9. Establish Healthy Boundaries:

- Learn to say no when necessary.
- Balance work and personal life to prevent burnout.

10. Seek Professional Support:

- Consult a therapist or counselor for guidance.
- Mental health professionals can provide tools and strategies for resilience.

11. Foster a Growth Mindset:

- Embrace challenges as opportunities to learn.
- See failures as stepping stones toward improvement.

12. Maintain a Healthy Lifestyle:

- Eat a balanced diet to support physical and mental health.
- Limit the consumption of substances that can negatively impact mental well-being.

13. Engage in Hobbies and Activities:

- Pursue activities that bring joy and fulfillment.
- Hobbies provide a healthy outlet for stress and creativity.

14. Practice Time Management:

- Prioritize tasks to reduce feelings of overwhelm.
- Break down tasks into manageable chunks for better focus.

15. Foster a Sense of Purpose:

- Identify your values and align your actions with them.
- Having a purpose enhances resilience during challenging times.

Incorporating these practical strategies into your daily life can contribute significantly to building and maintaining mental resilience. Consistent effort in these areas can help you navigate life's ups and downs with greater strength and adaptability.

Chapter Five

Lifestyle Habits for a Longer Life

In our fast-paced world, the pursuit of a longer and healthier life has become an increasingly prevalent goal. As individuals strive to enhance their overall well-being, the role of lifestyle habits in promoting longevity has taken center stage. This exploration delves into the intricate interplay between daily choices and their impact on longevity, shedding light on the significance of cultivating habits that extend beyond the conventional realms of diet and exercise. From the nuances of sleep hygiene to the influence of social connections, this examination aims to uncover the multifaceted tapestry of lifestyle choices that contribute to a more extended and fulfilling existence.

Within the fabric of longevity, this discussion will traverse diverse aspects, ranging from the physiological effects of regular physical activity to the psychological dimensions of stress management.

By examining the latest research findings and drawing insights from holistic approaches to well-being, we embark on a journey to unravel the secrets to a longer life. As we navigate the intricate web of lifestyle habits, the overarching theme emerges – a symbiotic relationship between conscious choices and the intricate machinery of the human body and mind. Join us in this exploration, as we navigate the terrain of lifestyle habits that hold the promise of not just adding years to life but adding life to years.

The Sleep Solution for Optimal Health

In our fast-paced world, where productivity is highly valued, the importance of sleep often takes a backseat. However, understanding and prioritizing sleep is crucial for achieving optimal health. This article explores the various aspects of the sleep solution and how it directly impacts our well-being.

The Science Behind Sleep

Sleep is not merely a state of rest; it is a complex physiological process essential for overall health. During sleep, the body undergoes crucial repair and maintenance activities. From consolidating memories to releasing growth hormones, each sleep stage plays a unique role in supporting physical and mental functions.

Quality vs. Quantity

It's not just about the hours spent in bed; the quality of sleep matters equally. Deep, uninterrupted sleep is essential for the body to enter restorative states. Factors such as sleep environment, mattress quality, and bedtime routine contribute significantly to the overall sleep experience.

Creating an Ideal Sleep Environment

Optimizing your sleep environment is a key component of the sleep solution. Keep your bedroom dark, cool, and quiet. Invest in a comfortable mattress and pillows that support proper spinal alignment. Have a consistent bed time.

The Impact of Technology

In the age of smartphones and constant connectivity, electronic devices can disrupt our circadian rhythm. Screens emit blue lights that interfere with the production of melatonin, a hormone crucial for sleep. Establishing a digital curfew and creating a tech-free zone in the bedroom can significantly improve sleep quality.

Nutrition and Sleep

How well you sleep can be affected by what you eat. Sleep patterns can be affected by taking caffeine and heavy meals close to bedtime. Conversely, certain foods, such as those rich in magnesium and tryptophan, can promote better sleep. Understanding the relationship between nutrition and sleep is a key aspect of the sleep solution.

Establishing a Consistent Sleep Schedule

Sleep-wake cycle is part of healthy routines we should adopt. Going to bed and waking up at the same time each day, even on weekends, helps regulate the body's internal clock. Consistency reinforces the natural circadian rhythm, promoting better sleep quality over time.

The Role of Stress Management

Stress and sleep are intricately connected. Insomnia can show up when chronic stress persists, also poor sleep can increase stress levels. Incorporating stress-reducing practices such as meditation, deep breathing, or gentle exercise into your daily routine can contribute to a more peaceful night's sleep.

Conclusion

Achieving optimal health involves recognizing the importance of sleep and implementing a comprehensive sleep solution. By understanding the science behind sleep, creating an ideal sleep environment, managing technology use, making informed nutritional choices, establishing a consistent sleep schedule, and practicing stress management, individuals can unlock the full potential of their physical and mental well-being. Prioritizing sleep is not a luxury; it is a necessity for a healthier and more fulfilling life.

Everyday Habits for Disease Defense and Longevity

In the pursuit of a long and healthy life, adopting practical habits is crucial. This guide explores actionable steps to fortify your defense against diseases and promote longevity.

1. Balanced Nutrition

A cornerstone of disease prevention is a well-balanced diet. Emphasize whole foods, rich in vitamins, minerals, and antioxidants. Incorporate diverse fruits, vegetables, lean proteins, and whole grains into your meals.

2. Regular Exercise

Engage in physical activity regularly. Aim for a mix of cardiovascular exercises, strength training, and flexibility exercises. Exercise not only strengthens your body but also boosts immune function and mental well-being.

3. Quality Sleep

Prioritize quality sleep for optimal health. Create a sleep-friendly environment, maintain a consistent sleep schedule, and ensure 7-9 hours of sleep per night. Quality sleep enhances immune function and supports overall well-being.

4. Hydration

Proper hydration is essential for bodily functions, including digestion, circulation, and temperature regulation.

5. Stress Management

Immune system can be weakened by chronic stress and it also contributes to different health issues.

Practice stress-reducing techniques such as meditation, deep breathing, or hobbies to foster emotional well-being.

6. Regular Health Check-ups

Regular health check-ups should be done regularly in order to detect potential issues early. Prevention and early intervention are key to maintaining good health.

7. Social Connections

Maintain meaningful social connections. Strong social ties contribute to emotional well-being, reducing the risk of mental health issues and providing a support system during challenging times.

8. Limiting Harmful Substances

Reduce or eliminate harmful substances such as tobacco and excessive alcohol from your lifestyle. These substances can contribute to various diseases and negatively impact overall health.

9. Sun Protection

Sunscreen should be used and sun safety measures should be practiced in order to protect your skin from harmful UV rays. This helps prevent skin cancer and promotes skin health.

10. Lifelong Learning

Engage in lifelong learning to keep your mind active and agile. Challenge your brain with new activities, hobbies, and educational pursuits to promote cognitive health.

Conclusion

By incorporating these practical habits into your daily life, you can significantly contribute to disease defense and enhance your chances of a long and healthy life. Consistency is key, and these habits work synergistically to create a foundation for overall well-being.

Conclusion

We have embarked on a transformative journey toward holistic well-being, discovering the intricate web of factors that contribute to a vibrant life. As we navigated the realms of metabolism, fat loss, and longevity, the tapestry of interconnected elements unfolded—nutrition, exercise, sleep, and mindfulness, weaving together a symphony of wellness. This comprehensive guide has not only equipped us with practical tools to enhance our metabolic vigor but has also illuminated the path to a healthier, more fulfilling existence.

Our exploration began with an understanding of metabolism as the metabolic engine driving the body's intricate processes. We delved into the symbiotic relationship between nutrition and metabolism, realizing the profound impact of balanced, nutrient-rich choices on our vitality. Through the chapters on targeted exercises and lifestyle adjustments, we harnessed the power to revitalize our bodies, shedding not just unwanted pounds but fostering resilience from within.

Fat loss, a common pursuit, was approached not merely as a cosmetic endeavor but as a pivotal step towards optimizing health. The book emphasized sustainable approaches, steering clear of quick fixes, and instead championing the enduring benefits of adopting habits that align with our body's natural rhythms.

The exploration of longevity provided a compelling conclusion, inviting us to consider the factors that extend the tapestry of our existence. From the science of aging to the art of mindful living, we unraveled the secrets to a prolonged and meaningful life. This journey, however, was not solely about extending our days but enriching each one with purpose, joy, and vitality.

As we bid farewell to these pages, let us carry forward the wisdom acquired. The true essence of revitalized health lies not in isolated interventions but in the harmonious integration of various elements—nutrition, fitness, mindfulness—into our daily lives. This is not a conclusion but a commencement—an invitation to embark on a lifelong journey of well-being, armed with the knowledge and tools to revitalize our health, embrace longevity, and savor the full spectrum of life's richness. May your path be illuminated by the glow of renewed vitality, and may "Revitalize Your Health" continue to serve as a guiding light on your ongoing adventure toward optimal well-being.